Meal Prep for Beginners

Recipes and Weekly Plans for Healthy,
Ready-to-Go Meals
Your Essential Guide To Losing Weight
And Saving Time - Delicious, Simple And
Healthy Meals To Prep and Go!

CONTENTS

Furthermore, the transmission, duplication, or reproduction of any of the following work including specific information will be considered an illegal act irrespective of if it is done electronically or in print. This extends to creating a secondary or tertiary copy of the work or a recorded copy and is only allowed with the express written consent from the Publisher. All additional right reserved.

A WEEK OF EASY MEALS
FOR BUSY PEOPLE

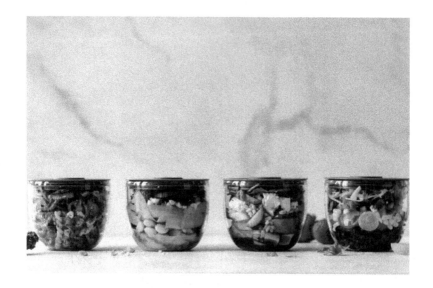

Would you like to know the best feeling on the planet? Looking into an ice chest of prepped nourishment on Sunday night, realizing you are good to go for snacks and even a few suppers for the week ahead. I affectionately consider it a "monster crowd" minute, twisting up like Smaug in self-satisfied fulfillment on your brilliant heap of ethically prepared meals.

So what gets you this enchantment minute? A Power Hour. Actually no, not the drinking game (despite the fact that if you need to toss that in, you do you). I'm discussing the hour or two when you turn on some music, sling on a cover, and power through the prep that will feed your week.

You see these prep minutes on Instagram; you couldn't want anything more than to do this as well. All things considered, welcome to Power Hour — our new arrangement where we give you how we plan and prep our own meals, pressing all that prep into about an hour or somewhat more. To kick things off, here's my very own Power Hour meal prep plan.

Here are my meal prep substances. I'm a mother of two children (2 and under); I work all day and don't have the opportunity to cook most evenings. So I consider meal prep as unadulterated need. I blast out however much as I can in my Sunday Power Hour so I can cook as meager as could be expected during the week. My scrumptious, large peered toward child is much additionally engaging on a Monday night, and she heads to sleep at 6:30, so I need constantly with her that I can get.

My significant other and I have a high resistance for rehashing meals. (Is this because we have a 8-month-old and a 2-year-old, who fill life with all the unexpected one's spirit pines for? SOMETHING TO PONDER!) So I cook large clusters of a couple of blend and-match supper choices, shop deliberately for snacks, and supplement these meals with takeout and the cooler.

My Meal Prep Goals

Breakfast: A major clump breakfast to last all week

Lunch: Lunches for me and my better half (five days).

Supper: Dinner for me and my better half (five to six days).

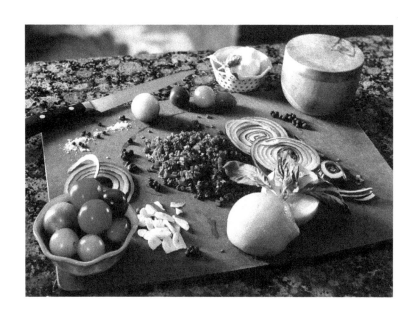

Nourishing Goals: We don't have any nourishment limitations. In any case, I search for high-volume yet generally low-calorie snacks with bunches of vegetables, and entire nourishment driven, straightforward suppers with a great deal of flavor.

Meal Prep Plan Snapshot

Feeds: Two to three individuals

Prep Time: About 2 hours

Meals Covered: About 80% (no end of the week meals)

Weeknight Cooking Required? Not so much. Simply warming.

My Meal Plan

Breakfast

Breakfast Egg Casserole with Sweet Potatoes, Arugula and Goat Cheese

Snacks

Bacon and Tomato Salad Swag: Soft-bubbled egg, bacon, goat cheddar, cherry tomatoes, vinegar shallots, stirred up every day with a pack of serving of mixed greens and some balsamic dressing.

Bite Lunch: My better half's favored method for having lunch. He takes a bento box loaded up with eating cheddar, berries, nuts, cut ringer pepper, and some moved lunch meat.

Blend and-Match Dinners

Broiled Chicken Thighs, Two Ways (Peanut Sauce and Shwarma-Spiced)

Bacon and Herb Couscous Salad

Nut Slaw

Cut Cucumbers

Cut Peaches

My Shopping List

These are the things I purchased or utilized for this meal prep plan.

Produce: Slaw blend, carrot slaw, cilantro, English cucumbers, berries, bananas, simmered peanuts, chime peppers, 3 boxes plate of mixed greens, 1 box infant arugula

Meat: 5 pounds boneless skinless chicken thighs, 1 pound bacon

Dairy: 2 dozen huge eggs, nearby entire milk, BabyBel cheddar, cheddar sticks, goat cheddar disintegrates

Wash room and Frozen: Peanut sauce (10-ounce bottle), solidified diced sweet potatoes (12-ounce sack), Outshine natural product popsicles

How I Get the Prep Done

Time to take out this prep! My Sunday evening prep list is as per the following (and we've made a convenient pinnable picture with the menu and prep list, if you're intrigued!).

Heat one full pound of bacon. I line a sheet container with foil and meal the bacon until fresh (adhere to these directions). When done, I channel off the fat and hack the bacon into reduced down pieces. Try not to wash the dish yet.

Cook the pearl couscous. In the interim, I heat chicken stock to the point of boiling and cook the pearl couscous (Trader Joe's Harvest Grains) until delicate, then spread it to cool on the bacon-spread sheet skillet.

Season the chicken thighs (two different ways!). While the bacon and couscous are cooking, I separate the chicken between two major prep bowls and season it. One half is prepared with a shwarma zest blend; the staying chicken is prepared with about portion of a jug of locally acquired nut sauce.

Cook the chicken thighs. When the bacon is out of the stove, I raise the temperature from 400°F to 450°F and cook the chicken thighs for 20 to 25 minutes or until rankled on the edges. When the chicken is done, I turn the broiler down to 375°F.

Blend and prepare the egg meal. While the thighs are cooking I prep the egg dish. I whisk 10 eggs with around 1/2 cups entire milk; season delicately with salt and pepper; and pour over a 12-ounce pack of still-solidified sweet potatoes, a large portion of a compartment of slashed arugula, and disintegrated goat cheddar. When the thighs are done, I put this in to heat for around 45 minutes or until puffed and set on top.

Make nut slaw. I hurl the slaw blend and destroyed carrots with the staying half container of nut sauce and a slashed pack of cilantro (leaves just), season to taste with salt, and top with squashed broiled peanuts.

Delicate bubble eggs. I delicate heat up twelve eggs utilizing our essential bubbled egg technique (I utilize a five-minute cook time for delicate however set yolks).

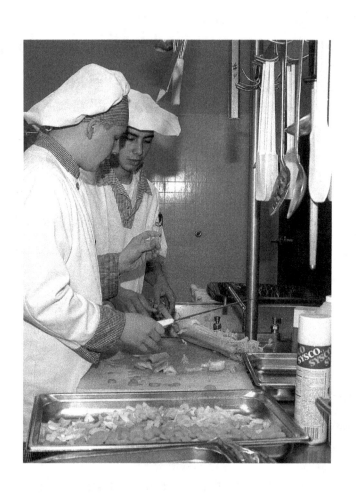

Make the pearl couscous serving of mixed greens. I lift the foil on the sheet dish to channel the couscous into a major blending bowl. I finely slash the rest of the arugula and hurl it with the couscous, alongside hacked herbs and about a large portion of the cleaved bacon. Taste and include salt and pepper.

Prep serving of mixed greens swag. Serving of mixed greens swag is everything except for the greens. I make up little boxes of cut cherry tomatoes, goat cheddar disintegrates, stripped delicate bubbled eggs, and some cut shallots hurled with vinegar.

Make up nibble lunch boxes. For my significant other (who makes me espresso each morning!), I make up lunch boxes of bunches of nibble y things like nuts, moved lunch meat, cheddar, cut ringer peppers, and berries.

What's more, that is it! Loads of cooking, yet once it's done and everything is refrigerated, I'm set for the week.

All out time: A little under two hours, if you don't check the breaks I took to nurture the infant and feed my baby lunch.

A Week of (Almost) Zero Weeknight Cooking

Here's the way all that prep transforms into seven days of very nearly zero cooking. Keep in mind — we have a high resistance for dullness in our meals.

Breakfast: My better half drives through the egg goulash (which he likewise flies into his lunch box on more than one occasion per week) and afterward goes to locally acquired yogurt and granola when it runs out. The little child eats solidified waffles, yogurt, organic product, or Cheerios — as her morning soul leads.

Lunch: I eat my serving of mixed greens swag boxes hurled with a colossal bowl of greens and some astounding tamari rosemary dressing from a neighborhood bistro. Heavenly. My significant other packs a nibble y lunch and on a couple of days seven days eats out with his graduate understudies or visiting staff. (His snacks may sound light, yet they're shockingly filling. He bicycles 10 miles every day and these appear to hold him well.)

The little child eats edamame from the cooler, cheddar, pasta, turkey meatballs from the cooler, and a not-insignificant-amount of PB&J.

Supper: I travel one night this week and eat air terminal sushi (why truly, I live on the edge, much obliged). The remainder of the evenings, I heat up the grill and rapidly cook some chicken thighs to warm them and include some additional flavor. Then we eat the nut sauce chicken with nut slaw, or the shwarma-spiced chicken with the couscous plate of mixed greens — likely sitting on the floor with the infant and little child. The little child eats something nibble y like veggies from the cooler, saltines, sweet potato fries with ketchup, cheddar, and — consistently — an Outshine organic product Popsicle. We as a whole offer peach cuts and perhaps a few cucumbers with farm dressing.

Afterward, I strike the cooler for a chomp of Jeni's. Because a decent meal-prepper merits her prize.

BEAN RECIPES ARE MEAL PREP MIRACLES

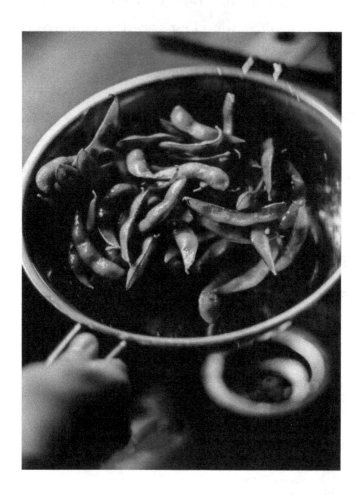

We've touted the advantages of keeping a couple of jars of beans reserved in the wash room and working this modest, protein-rich staple into your meal plan. In any case, where it truly proves to be useful is when you're meal prepping for the week ahead. Not exclusively does this generous wash room staple keep its toothsome surface and hold up as time goes on, however beans likewise often get considerably more flavor for a long time. Here are 10 simple plans to work beans into your meal prep schedule.

1. Swiss Chard with Garbanzo Beans

Regardless of whether you eat it warm or cooled, this Italian interpretation of beans and greens will undoubtedly turn into a standard expansion to your meal prep session. The plans calls for chickpeas, yet you can swap in a canned beans. Eat it all alone, beat with an egg, spooned over toast, or stuffed into a pita or prepared potato.

We like to put Swiss chard on the table as the meal's vegetable because, as other verdant greens, it has bunches of dietary advantages. Notwithstanding, it tends to be somewhat insipid so we include a couple of different fixings like pancetta, shallot, and garbanzo beans to give it a lift. As the beans cook, they separate a little to thicken the cooking juices. We likewise like this piled onto bruschetta as an appetizer or light lunch.

An Italian Take on Beans and Greens

This straightforward dish takes the great mix of beans and greens and puts an Italian turn on things. Hacked shallots and salty, lavishly enhanced pancetta add interest to healthy sautéed Swiss chard and substantial chickpeas, while a touch of red pepper drops include the perfect amout of zest. This dish makes for one healthy lunch or light supper all alone, however can likewise play side dish to cooks or become a simple canapé when heaped on bruschetta. Remains likewise keep quite well, so you can dive into it today and afterward appreciate it a couple of different ways over the next days.

Swiss Chard with Garbanzo Beans (Bietole e ceci)
SERVES
4 to 6
Fixings
2 pounds Swiss chard, ideally rainbow chard
2 tablespoons extra-virgin olive oil
2 ounces pancetta, cut into 1/4-inch dice (around 1/2 cup)
2 tablespoons finely slashed shallot
Squeeze red pepper drops
1 can garbanzo beans, depleted and flushed
Salt

Naturally ground dark pepper

Guidelines

Wash the chard leaves and stems well in an enormous sink of cold water. Lift the chard out of the water, leaving the coarseness at the base of the sink. Shake off the overabundance water, yet don't dry the chard.

Tear the stems from the leaves and hack the stems across into 1/2-inch pieces; put in a safe spot. Stack the leaves and coarsely cleave them. Keep the stems and leaves independent.

Warmth the oil in a huge skillet over medium-high warmth. Include the pancetta and cook until fresh and carmelized, around 3 minutes. Mix in the shallot and red pepper pieces and cook, mixing often, until the shallot softens, around 2 minutes.

Include the chard stems and beans. Cook, blending at times, until the stems soften, around 4 minutes. Mix in the leaves a bunch at once until shriveled. Spread and cook, blending infrequently, until the chard is delicate, around 5 minutes. Taste and season with salt and pepper as required. Serve hot.

Formula NOTES

Capacity: Leftovers can be put away in a hermetically sealed compartment in the cooler for as long as 5 days.

Make ahead: The chard can be washed and slice as long as 1 day ahead and put away in the fridge.

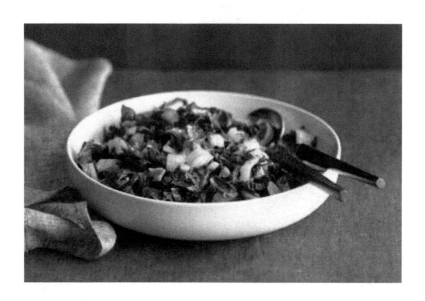

2. Marinated White Beans

The most great thing about marinated beans is that they get increasingly more flavor each day. This is an extraordinary one to meal prep if you need a lunch alternative that doesn't need to be refrigerated.

When absorbed garlic and shallot-implanted olive oil and hurled with heaps of crisp herbs, stout white beans change into a tasty multi-reason dish. Carry them to a cookout, heap them onto thick cuts of toast for supper, or hurl with cooked grains for a healthy and fulfilling lunch.

This is only the sort of staple worth having close by throughout the entire summer, when light, no-cook meals are the need and easy eating is at the forefront of everybody's thoughts. These beans let you quit stressing over what's for lunch or supper with the goal that you can invest more energy relaxing on the patio.

An Easy, No-Cook Recipe That Gets Better as It Sits

What makes these beans additional uncommon is that their flavor improves the more they sit. In the wake of combining everything, you'll toss them in the ice chest to absorb all the rich olive oil and new herb enhance. Following a couple of days, you'll come back to a multipurpose dish that is light, crisp, and fulfilling.

The beans are magnificent spooned onto toast or used to beef up a plate of mixed greens, yet I particularly love them hurled with cooked farro or dark colored rice, because the garlicky oil covers each grain. They'd likewise be a decent backup to barbecued steak or frankfurters. Or on the other hand, you could simply feel free to eat them by the spoonful — they're actually that great.

Marinated White Beans

MAKES

3 cups

SERVES

4 to 6

PREP TIME:

10 minutes

Fixings

1/3 cup olive oil

Finely ground pizzazz of 1 medium lemon

Juice of 1 medium lemon

1 medium shallot, diced (around 1/4 cup)

1 clove garlic, ground or minced

1/2 teaspoon fit salt, in addition to additional as required

Newly ground dark pepper

2 (15-ounce) jars cannellini beans, depleted and washed

1/3 cup hacked new level leaf parsley leaves

1/4 cup hacked new oregano leaves

Directions

Spot the olive oil, lemon get-up-and-go and squeeze, shallot, garlic, salt, and scarcely any liberal toils of dark pepper in an enormous bowl and rush to consolidate. Include the white beans, parsley, and oregano and hurl to consolidate. Taste and season with progressively salt and pepper as required.

Cover and refrigerate for in any event 20 minutes or medium-term. Let come to room temperature before serving.

Formula NOTES

Make ahead: These beans show signs of improvement with time, so don't hesitate to make them as long as 2 days early and store in the icebox.

Serving recommendations: The beans can be delighted in as seems to be, heaped on toast, prepared with cooked grains, or served over plates of mixed greens.

Capacity: Leftovers can be put away in an impenetrable holder in the fridge for as long as 3 days.

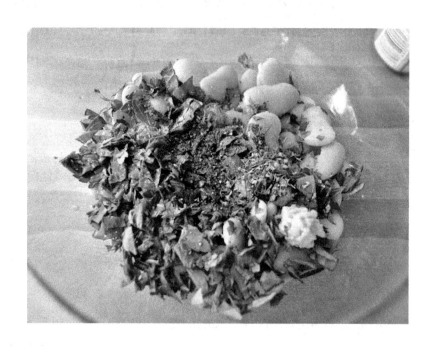

3. Dark Bean Corn Salsa

Stuff this thick salsa in a delicate flour tortilla with some sharp cream and guac, wrap it up, and you have a supper that meets up in negligible minutes. It's additionally healthy enough to be the protein-stuffed fundamental in a burrito bowl.

If there was ever an opportunity to keep tortilla chips supplied in your wash room, it's currently. When hurled with lime juice, fiery chipotles, and crisp cilantro, a humble jar of dark beans and an ear of new summer corn are changed into a strong, full-seasoned salsa you'll need to eat with all the fixings. It's both a group satisfying plunge and the base of a no-cook summer dinner.

The Do-Anything, Go-Anywhere Salsa

As a matter of first importance, similar to any salsa, this one is a group satisfying gathering plunge. In any case, that is only one of the numerous caps it wears. On evenings you don't want to cook (or it's essentially excessively blistering), spoon this generous salsa into a delicate tortilla, top with a bit of Greek yogurt and guac, and you have a no-muss, straightforward meal on your hands. Past that, spoon it over barbecued chicken, fish, or pork slashes, or make it the star of your next burrito bowl.

This formula calls for one loading cup of corn parts, which is just about the sum you'll get from a normal estimated ear of corn. When crisp corn is in season, you'll need to utilize it in this salsa, yet defrosted solidified corn can be subbed in different seasons. The surface of solidified pieces is somewhat gentler, however you can anticipate a similar delightful outcome.

Dark Bean and Corn Salsa

MAKES

around 3 cups

SERVES

Makes 3 cups

PREP TIME:

10 minutes to 15 minutes

Fixings

1 (15.5-ounce) can dark beans, depleted and flushed

1 storing cup crisp or defrosted solidified corn portions (if utilizing new, around 1 ear)

1 medium plum tomato, seeded and diced

1/2 little red onion, diced

1/2 cup finely slashed crisp cilantro leaves and delicate stems

1 canned chipotle chile in adobo sauce, finely slashed, in addition to 2 tablespoons of the adobo sauce

Juice from 1/2 medium lime

1/4 teaspoon legitimate salt

Directions

Spot every one of the fixings in a medium bowl and mix to consolidate. Cover and refrigerate in any event 30 minutes before serving to enable the flavors to merge.

Formula NOTES

Capacity: Leftovers can be refrigerated in a concealed compartment for to multi week.

Without gluten: For sans gluten salsa, ensure the brand of chipotles in adobo sauce is sans wheat.

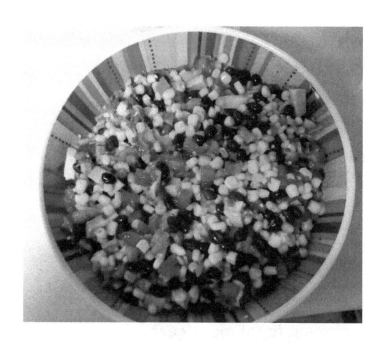

4. Mixed Chickpea and Spinach Pitas

Regardless of what meal of the day you serve these pitas, you can't turn out badly. Cook the chickpea filling and amass the pitas during meal prep, then reserve then in the cooler for some other time.

For a vegetarian breakfast sandwich that self-control you through the morning, look to this pita pocket loaded down with a mix of spiced chickpeas and sautéed veggies. It's prepared ahead of time, then reserved in the cooler, fit to be warmed in the broiler while you buzz through your morning schedule.

Getting the Right Mix of Textures

To get the correct surface for this filling, a large portion of the chickpeas are pounded before they are sautéed in coconut oil alongside cumin, turmeric, garlic powder, and veggies like spinach and red chime peppers.

Make-Ahead Breakfast Sandwiches

Made in a major clump, these cooler well-disposed breakfast sandwiches are your answer for a simple and fulfilling sweltering breakfast on even the most furious weekday mornings. Because you're placing in the work to prepare breakfast ahead of time, you have the right to benefit from your endeavors. Every one of these sandwiches will take you through well over seven days of morning meals.

Mixed Chickpea and Spinach Pitas

MAKES

12

Fixings

6 (15-ounce) jars garbanzo beans, depleted and flushed

1/4 cup coconut oil

1 medium onion, diced

2 medium red ringer peppers, cored, seeded, and diced

2 1/2 teaspoons ground cumin

2 teaspoons ground turmeric

1 teaspoon garlic powder (no salt)

1 teaspoon fit salt

6 cups infant spinach, coarsely slashed

6 standard measured pita breads, divided to shape half moons

Guidelines

Add half of the chickpeas to a nourishment processor fitted with the edge connection and heartbeat until separated yet not puréed. (On the other hand, place in an enormous bowl and pound with a fork.) Set aside.

Warmth the coconut oil in a 12-inch (or bigger), high-sided skillet over medium warmth until shining. Include the onions, mix to cover with the oil, and cook until delicate, 4 to 5 minutes. Mix in the ringer peppers, cumin, turmeric, garlic powder, and salt, and cook until the peppers are delicate, around 4 minutes.

Include the squashed and entire chickpeas, mix to join, and cook until they start to soften, around 5 minutes. Mix in the spinach, cooking just until withered, around 3 minutes. Expel the container from the warmth.

To serve promptly, isolate the chickpea blend between the pitas, filling every half with 3/4 to 1 cup of the blend.

Warming:

If not serving quickly, let the chickpea blend cool totally before filling, then wrap every pita half firmly in aluminum foil. Refrigerate or stop in resealable plastic packs. Warm revealed in a 325°F standard or toaster broiler until warmed through, around 20 minutes if refrigerated or around 30 minutes if solidified.

Formula NOTES

Capacity: The stuffed pitas enveloped by foil can be put away in resealable plastic sacks in the icebox for as long as 3 days or in the cooler for as long as 3 months.

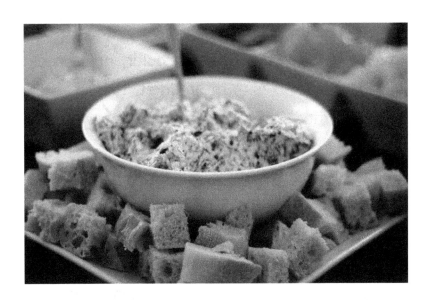

5. Simple Slow Cooker Bean Soup

Start with a pound of a beans or combo of beans and incline toward your moderate cooker to breathe life into this delightful soup.

Smoked ham or turkey bones are one of the most misjudged (also simplest) approaches to include profound, appetizing flavor to anything that you're making — and this soup is no exemption. Get them from the butcher or out of your cooler, get a pack of those dried bean mixes in the market, toss everything else into the moderate cooker with some water, and approach your day.

When you return, the water will mysteriously change into a thick, soothing stock that holds delicate beans, vegetables, and slivers of delectable, smoky meat.

Smoked Meat = Flavor

The sort of smoked meat you use here is actually very adaptable: turkey or ham legs give you the most meat, however ham sells wings still contribute huge amounts of flavor and smokiness. It additionally implies that the soup can be made with water and not stock.

Bean Blend, Not Bean Soup

Notably, there are the same number of dried bean mixes out there as there are brands. Each brand appears to have their own mix, from a couple of different sorts of beans to up to 15! Simply get what's accessible (and don't stress if the bundle isn't actually a pound) — however ensure it is anything but a soup mix that has included dried vegetables, flavors, or herbs to it.

There's additionally no compelling reason to douse the beans already, as the long stretch in the moderate cooker does all the difficult work to yield delicate, tasty beans. A modest of spoonful of apple juice vinegar toward the end carries sharpness and center to throughout the entire the stewed flavors, so don't avoid the progression — you'll be flabbergasted at the difference it makes!

Simple Slow Cooker Bean Soup

MAKES

around 2 1/2 quarts

SERVES

6 to 8

Fixings

For the soup:

8 cups (2 quarts) water

1 sack (around 1 pound) dried bean mix (not bean soup mix)

1/2 to 2 pounds smoked ham pawns, ham bone, or turkey leg or wings

1 medium yellow onion, little bones

1 cup stripped and diced carrots

1 cup diced celery

1/2 teaspoon dried thyme

1 straight leaf

1/4 teaspoon crisply ground dark pepper

To wrap up:

Apple juice vinegar

Salt

Coarsely slashed crisp parsley leaves

Guidelines

Spot all the soup fixings in a 6-quart or bigger moderate cooker, ensuring everything is submerged in water. Spread and cook on the LOW setting until the beans are delicate, 8 to 10 hours.

Utilizing tongs, move the ham or turkey onto a cutting board and let cool marginally. In the interim, mix the soup, taste, and season with salt and vinegar (1/2 teaspoon of vinegar at once) as required. Expel the meat from the bones, shred, and mix again into the soup (dispose of the bones and any skin). If you need a more slender soup, include water as required. Serve bested with parsley.

Formula NOTES

Capacity: Leftovers can be put away in a hermetically sealed compartment in the fridge for as long as 5 days or solidified for as long as 3 months.

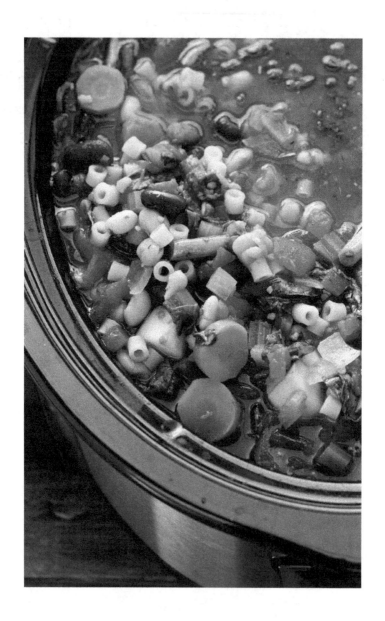

6. Tomato and Feta White Bean Salad

When it comes to servings of mixed greens, probably the best wagered when getting a head start is plans that utilization beans as a base. They get more flavor for a long time and don't shrivel or get soaked. Quinoa, farro, destroyed chicken, or a couple of portions of extra steak are a simple method to build it up.

Here's a straightforward yet fulfilling plate of mixed greens to make for supper this evening. If you have two or three jars of white beans in your wash room, you're as of now most of the way there. Channel the beans and hurl in the same number of succulent, in-season cherry tomatoes as you can fit in the bowl; include a couple of large bunches of tart, salty feta and a lot of hacked new parsley and oregano; and afterward dress the entire chaos in a sharp, sweet-smelling shallot vinaigrette. The outcome is a flavor-stuffed plate of mixed greens that feels healthy yet still light and new enough to fit the season.

A Fast Salad for Slow Summer Days

This formula meets up in only a couple of moments, which guarantees that it wins on occupied weeknights. It's very primary course-commendable if you're needing a filling meatless (and sans gluten) supper or lunch, yet it additionally functions admirably as a side. Pair it with flame broiled meat or fish or tote it to your next potluck to join the spread of sides for the group's burgers and sausages. Despite how you decide to appreciate it, it's certain to turn into a late spring backup.

Tomato and Feta White Bean Salad

SERVES

2 to 4; makes around 5 cups

Fixings

2 tablespoons olive oil

1 tablespoon red wine vinegar

1 teaspoon minced shallot

Fit salt

Naturally ground dark pepper

1 (15-ounce) can white beans, depleted and flushed

1 16 ounces cherry or grape tomatoes (around 2 cups), split

4 ounces feta cheddar, disintegrated (around 1 cup)

1/2 cup coarsely hacked crisp parsley leaves

2 tablespoons hacked crisp oregano leaves

Directions

Whisk the oil, vinegar, shallot, a major touch of salt, and a couple of liberal toils of dark pepper together in an enormous bowl. Include the beans, tomatoes, feta, parsley, and oregano and hurl to join. Taste and include increasingly salt and pepper as required.

Formula NOTES

Capacity: Leftovers can be put away in a sealed shut holder in the fridge for as long as 3 days.

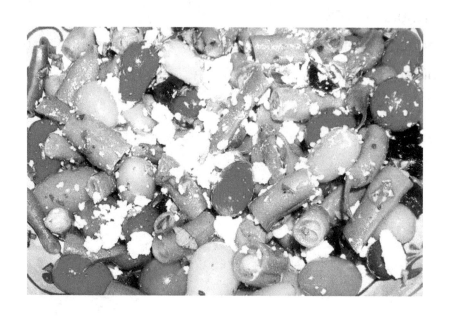

7. Kidney Bean and Coconut Curry

If you've been saving kidney beans for stew, this is another healthy, soothing approach to give then something to do. Canned beans can be utilized instead of dried to chop down the prep time. Remember to make a pot of rice while the curry is stewing to balance your meal prep.

Healthy and veggie lover? Is it conceivable? Indeed, obviously! We pulled plans from a couple of veggie lover cookbooks hitting the market this year and solicited one from our nourishment picture takers and beauticians, Maria Siriano, who happens to be vegetarian, for her musings on the plans.

Veggie lover: The Cookbook by Jean-Christian Jury is a visit de power of vegetarian food propelled by the culinary conventions from each edge of the globe. This cookbook is a piece of the Phaidon culinary book of scriptures arrangement so it's a major one, pressing in around 500 plans highlighting a scope of fixings and strategies. We adored the kidney bean and coconut curry, a formula hailing from the culinary customs of Chad — despite the fact that you'll discover comparative dishes of beans stewed in coconut milk all through the world — for its effortlessness and clear flavors.

Kidney Bean and Coconut Curry

SERVES

4

Fixings

2 cups dried kidney beans, absorbed water medium-term

2 tablespoons vegetable oil

2 medium red onions, hacked

2 medium tomatoes, hacked

2 cups coconut milk

1 teaspoon ground cardamom

2 cloves garlic, squashed

1 tablespoon yellow curry powder

---

1 medium jalapeño, seeded and finely hacked

Salt

2 tablespoon coarsely hacked new cilantro

Cooked basmati or jasmine rice, for serving

Directions

Channel and wash the drenched kidney beans. Fill a huge pot with enough water to cover the kidney beans and heat to the point of boiling. Include the beans and stew over low warmth until delicate, around 60 minutes. Channel and put in a safe spot.

Warmth the oil in a similar pot over medium warmth until gleaming. Include the onion and cook, blending incidentally, until softened, 3 to 4 minutes. Include the tomatoes and cook for 4 to 5 minutes. Include the held kidney beans, coconut milk, cardamom, garlic, curry powder, and jalapeño. Season with salt, mix to consolidate, and stew over low warmth for 20 minutes. Topping with the cilantro and present with rice.

Formula NOTES

Capacity: Leftovers can be put away in a hermetically sealed compartment in the fridge for as long as multi week.

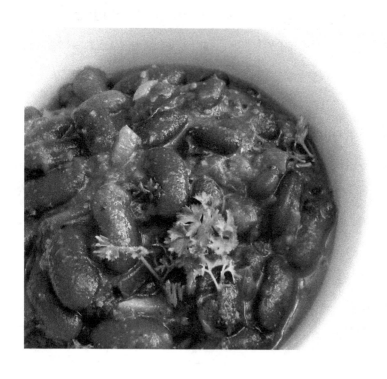

8. Chickpea and Cheddar Quesadillas

If your lunch battle includes thinking of veggie-accommodating alternatives that are filling, simple to make ahead, and a breeze to eat at your work area, this wrapped quesadilla loaded down with cumin-scented chickpeas, gooey softened cheddar, and scallions was made in view of you.

If your lunch battle includes thinking of veggie-accommodating choices that are filling, simple to make ahead, and a breeze to eat at your work area, this wrapped quesadilla loaded down with cumin-scented chickpeas, gooey dissolved cheddar, and scallions was made in light of you.

Pressing Quesadillas for Lunch

To make these quesadillas work area lunch-accommodating, we dumped the great wedge-cut quesadilla for a system that keeps the chickpeas and cheddar solidly settled in a completely shut tortilla: the wrapped quesadilla. When amassing, the fixings are layered in the focal point of the tortilla, then the edges of the tortilla are shut over the filling in five folds. It's much simpler to collect than it may sound, and once you get moving you'll perceive that it is so natural to get.

This make-ahead lunch will keep going for around three days in the ice chest or as long as a quarter of a year in the cooler. Keep them exclusively enveloped by foil and they can go directly from the refrigerator or cooler into the toaster (or customary) stove. It's ideal to skip microwave warming since it leaves the quesadilla chewy and soaked.

Chickpea and Cheddar Quesadillas

MAKES

4

Fixings

2 (15-ounce) jars garbanzo beans, depleted and washed, partitioned

1 tablespoon olive oil

1 little yellow onion, diced

1 clove garlic, finely hacked

1/2 teaspoons ground cumin

1 teaspoon stew powder

3/4 teaspoon legitimate salt

4 huge (9-to 10-inch) flour tortillas

2 cups destroyed cheddar

3 medium scallions, green parts just, daintily cut

Discretionary fixings:

Salsa, guacamole, acrid cream, Mexican hot sauce

Directions

Add half of the chickpeas to a nourishment processor fitted with the sharp edge connection and heartbeat until separated however not puréed. (On the other hand, place in a huge bowl and pound with a fork.) Set aside.

Warmth the oil in a huge griddle (at any rate 10 inches) over medium-high warmth until shining. Include the onion, mix to cover with the oil, and cook, blending periodically, until delicate, around 5 minutes. Include the entire and pounded chickpeas, garlic, cumin, bean stew powder, and salt. Cook, blending incidentally, for 3 minutes. Expel from the warmth.

Amass the quesadillas:

Spot the tortillas on a work surface. Top every tortilla with 1/4 cup of cheddar. Gap the chickpea blend among the tortillas, spreading into an even layer yet leaving a 1/2-inch fringe. Sprinkle the rest of the cheddar over top of the chickpeas, then top each with scallions.

To overlap the quesadillas, overlay the highest point of the tortilla down over the filling to the inside. Holding that piece down and working clockwise, keep collapsing the remainder of the tortilla towards the center until the filling is totally secured (you will have around 5 folds). Cautiously flip the quesadilla over and rehash with the rest of the tortillas.

Warmth a huge skillet or frying pan over medium warmth. Include the quesadillas (the same number of as will fit in a solitary layer), collapsed side down. Cook until carmelized, 4 to 5 minutes for every side. Rehash as required until every one of the quesadillas are cooked.

Warming:

If not serving quickly, let cool totally and wrap every quesadilla firmly in aluminum foil. Refrigerate or stop in resealable plastic sacks. Warm revealed in a 325°F standard or toaster stove until warmed through, around 15 minutes if refrigerated, or around 25 minutes if solidified. Microwaving isn't prescribed, as the quesadillas will be spongy.

Formula NOTES

Capacity: The foil-wrapped quesadillas can be put away in a resealable plastic sack in the fridge for as long as 3 days or in the cooler for as long as 3 months.

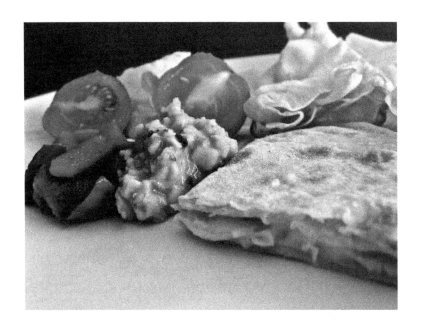

9. Dark Bean Burgers with Chipotle Ketchup

While veggie burgers are commonly simple to make (like this one), they require more prep than feels possible on a weeknight, which makes them an ideal meal prep up-and-comer. Truth be told, I prescribe making a twofold group and solidifying the remainder of later.

You don't need to be a veggie lover to adore these healthy, delightful meatless burgers. (You can, be that as it may, give them significantly increasingly appetizing substantiality by including cleaved sautéed shiitake or cremini mushrooms to the blend before framing the burgers).

Furthermore, definitely, make a twofold cluster of the ketchup — you'll locate a million uses for it, and it keeps well in the fridge for seven days.

These burgers can be made ahead of time and delicately warmed in a low broiler or on a low flame broil away from the immediate warmth. (Spot them on a bit of oiled foil and not straightforwardly on the barbecue rack.)

Serve this meal with:

Barbecued Guacamole

Macaroni Salad

Asian Cabbage, Carrot, and Peanut Slaw

Sicilian Greens

Strawberry Cheesecake Tart

Dark Bean Burgers with Chipotle Ketchup

SERVES

4

Fixings

For the burgers:

1 enormous egg, daintily beaten

2 (15.5-ounce) jars low-sodium dark beans, depleted and flushed

1/3 cup dry bread morsels

1/4 cup finely slashed red onion

1/4 cup slashed cilantro

3 tablespoons canola mayonnaise

1 teaspoon ground cumin

For the chipotle ketchup:

1/2 cup ketchup

1/2 chipotle in adobo, minced (around 1 tablespoon), or to taste

1 teaspoon lime juice

1 teaspoon nectar

1/4 teaspoon bean stew powder

To make the burgers:

2 tablespoons olive oil

4 Hawaiian sweet burger moves, split and toasted

Directions

Make the bean burger patties:

Join the egg and beans in an enormous bowl and crush them into pieces with a potato masher or huge fork. (Every one of the beans ought to be separated, however there should in any case be pieces obvious.) Add the breadcrumbs, onion, cilantro, mayonnaise, and cumin; mix to completely consolidate. Structure into four 1/2-inch-thick patties.

Make the ketchup:

Join the ketchup, chipotle, lime juice, nectar, cumin, and bean stew powder in a bowl, and put in a safe spot.

Cook the burgers:

Warmth the oil in a huge nonstick skillet over medium-high. Include the patties and cook until fresh and warmed through, around 4 minutes for every side. Serve on the moves bested with the chipotle ketchup.

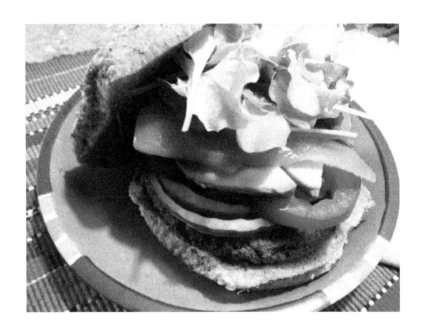

10. Chickpea Nuggets

Produced using a bunch of wash room staples, those without meat pieces can be absolutely prepped and prepared during your meal prep session, the warmed in the stove before supper.

Getting children to attempt new nourishments is basically an activity in advertising. A valid example: When I made falafel for supper one night, I called them chickpea pieces rather than falafel and my youngsters ate them straight up. They requested chickpea pieces again and it got my mind beating with a thought for a real chickpea chunk formula — one with every one of the flavors and surfaces of chicken tenders, yet prepared and sans egg.

These chickpea chunks look like chicken tenders, however are veggie lover and require just six storeroom staples. What's more, they're absolutely scrumptious!

Plant-Powered and Pantry-Friendly

Two storeroom staples are liable for transforming a humble jar of chickpeas into pieces: moved oats and the fluid from the chickpeas themselves (otherwise known as aquafaba). Crushing the oats into flour makes them practically imperceptible in the chunks, yet their expansion makes these pieces a total protein and all the more filling. The chickpea fluid goes about as a substitution for eggs, which would ordinarily hold this kind of piece elective together.

Toasting the panko breadcrumbs before covering the pieces gives the chickpea chunks a more extravagant shade, yet in addition includes flavor and heaps of crunchy surface. This single step gives the hallucination of chicken strips rather than chickpea pieces.

While this formula may have happened as expected for my youngsters, I concede that these delectable chunks were delighted in by grown-ups also. You can without much of a stretch appreciate them as you may a falafel (enveloped by pita and showered with yogurt), over a serving of mixed greens, or like the great child nourishment we love, with a lot of ketchup for plunging.

Chickpea Nuggets

SERVES

4

Fixings

———

1/2 cup panko or without gluten breadcrumbs

1/2 cup moved oats

1 (15-ounce) can garbanzo beans (don't deplete)

1 teaspoon fit salt

1/2 teaspoon garlic powder (no salt)

1/2 teaspoon onion powder (no salt)

Guidelines

Mastermind a rack in the stove and warmth to 375°F.

Spot the panko on a rimmed preparing sheet and heat until toasted and brilliant dark colored, around 5 minutes. Move to a bowl and put aside to cool while preparing the pieces. Line the preparing sheet with material paper.

Spot the oats in a nourishment processor fitted with the cutting edge connection and procedure into a fine flour. Move to a huge bowl and save the nourishment processor.

Channel the chickpeas over a bowl or estimating cup, then spare the chickpeas and 1/4 cup of the fluid. Spot the chickpeas into the nourishment processor; include the salt, garlic, and onion powder; and heartbeat until brittle. Keep blend in the nourishment processor.

Whisk 1/4 cup of the chickpea fluid in a little blending bowl until frothy. Include the frothy chickpea fluid and 1/2 cup of the oat flour to the nourishment processor. Heartbeat until the blend frames a ball. You may have a little oat flour extra, which you can add to the chickpea blend 1 tablespoon at once if the blend is free. Separation the chickpea blend into 12 equivalent parts and shape every one into a chunk. Coat every chunk totally in the toasted panko and spot on the material lined heating sheet.

Prepare until fresh, 15 to 20 minutes. Serve warm with your most loved plunging sauce.

Formula NOTES

Without gluten: These pieces can be made sans gluten by utilizing sans gluten oats and subbing sans gluten breadcrumbs for the panko.

Capacity: Leftovers can be put away in a hermetically sealed compartment in the fridge for as long as 5 days.

STEP BY STEP INSTRUCTIONS TO COOK CHICKEN BREAST IN THE INSTANT POT

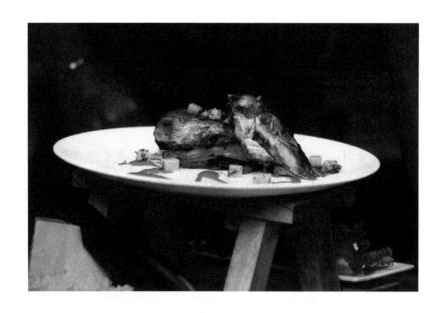

The main thing I propose making in your spic and span electric weight cooker is hard-cooked eggs (truly, so natural to strip). The second? Fundamental chicken bosom! This supper staple prepares up consummately every time in the Instant Pot. You can go for firm yet succulent chicken for cubing, or let it cook somewhat longer for delicate destroyed chicken.

Moment Pot chicken bosom is additionally as quick for meal prep (hi, more stove space!) all things considered for weeknight suppers. You can even cook solidified chicken bosom thusly while you make sense of the remainder of supper. Prepared for the basic steamed chicken bosom system you'll use again and again?

Essential, Not Boring, Chicken Breast in the Instant Pot

There are a ton of approaches to cook chicken in the electric weight cooker, yet this strategy is specifically for plain chicken bosom that you can use as meal prep for building servings of mixed greens and grain bowls or for utilizing in plans that call for cooked chicken. (This chicken plate of mixed greens rings a bell.)

Indeed, this formula underneath is simply chicken, salt, and chicken juices or water, however you can absolutely include your very own flavors before cooking with dry zest rubs or citrus, or spruce up the cooked chicken with sauces or salsas. There's no compelling reason to change the cooking time when including any of these for enhance.

It will take around 12 minutes for the Instant Pot to come up to temperature and afterward another 10 to 15 minutes of cook time. Contingent upon how you'd like your chicken concocted, you'd signify five minutes of normal discharge time. Your all out cook time, including prep? Thirty minutes. Could it be any more obvious? Better, quicker meal prep is standing by!

Would i be able to cook solidified chicken bosoms in the Instant Pot?

Truly! This technique works with solidified chicken also. Simply plan for solidified bosoms to take more time to come to temperature — around two to five minutes extra relying upon the quantity of bosoms. The cook time under strain doesn't change, yet it extends the measure of time it takes the pot to come up to strain to around 15 minutes

Utilize the trivet or steamer crate.

We're not heating up these bosoms, but instead constrain steaming them to guarantee they're succulent, so you need the bosoms to sit over the cooking fluid. I've utilized both the trivet that accompanies the pot and a collapsing steamer container with a similar extraordinary outcomes.

What is your chicken objective?

I need my chicken to be firm, and simple to dice: For firm, chicken serving of mixed greens prepared bosoms, you'll need to go for a 10-minute cook time however utilize a fast arrival of strain to keep the bosoms succulent and not overcooked.

I need delicate, destroyed chicken: For chicken that can be destroyed with a fork, keep the weight on somewhat longer by utilizing common discharge for five minutes following a 15-minute cook time.

Try not to hurl the juices! Whatever you do, don't dump the stock (or water) you utilized for steaming — it didn't lose any flavor, in certainty it increased a few, and you can utilize it to transform your chicken into soup or even to update your lunch ramen.

Step by step instructions to Cook Chicken Breast in the Instant Pot

SERVES

4 to 6

Fixings

3 pounds crisp or solidified boneless, skinless chicken bosoms (around 4 huge bosoms)

1 teaspoon fit salt

1 cup low-sodium chicken juices or water

Hardware

Electric weight cooker

Weight cooker rack or steamer container

Estimating cups and spoons

Guidelines

Mastermind the chicken, salt, and water in the electric weight cooker. Set the Instant Pot's trivet or a steamer bin inside the supplement of a 6-quart or bigger Instant Pot or electric weight cooker. Season the chicken with the salt and set on the trivet. Pour the chicken soup or water over the chicken.

For impeccably delicious chicken bosom: Cook the chicken on HIGH weight for 10 minutes and speedy discharge the weight. Seal the cooker and ensure the weight valve is shut. Set to HIGH weight for 10 minutes. For new chicken, it will take around 10 minutes to come to pressure. Anticipate that solidified chicken should take 12 to 15 minutes to come up to weight. When the 10-minute concoct time is, do a snappy arrival of the weight.

For destroyed chicken: Cook the chicken on HIGH weight for 15 minutes and characteristic discharge for 5 minutes. For chicken that shreds effectively with a fork, you'll need only a couple of more minutes of cooking and normal discharge. Seal the cooker and ensure the weight valve is shut. Set to HIGH weight for 15 minutes. For new chicken, the cooker will take around 10 minutes to come to pressure. Anticipate that solidified chicken should take 12 to 15 minutes to come to pressure. When the brief concoct time is, do a characteristic arrival of weight for 5 minutes before snappy discharging any residual weight.

Discharge remaining weight, evacuate and serve or use for some time later. Promptly move the chicken to a cutting board. If saving the prepared chicken for meals consistently, store the bosoms entire to keep them sodden. Hack or shred the chicken as wanted for prompt use in different plans. Save the stock for soups and cooking grains.

Formula NOTES

Solidified chicken: This strategy functions admirably with solidified chicken also, simply remember that solidified bosoms cool the cooker's addition and make for a more drawn out cooker time, as the weight cooker needs more opportunity to come to pressure.

Capacity: Cooked chicken can be put away in a hermetically sealed holder in the fridge for as long as 4 days.

THE MOST EFFECTIVE METHOD TO ROAST A CHICKEN

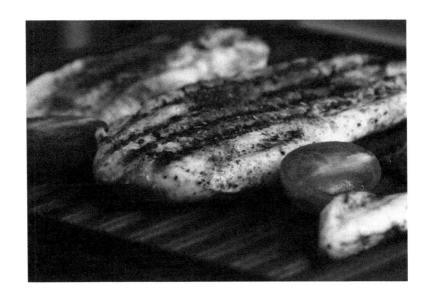

Figuring out how to broil a chicken has a guarantee past what most plans convey. Truly, a chicken will become supper, extra lunch, and ideally soup, yet a dish chicken additionally guarantees a night went through in the kitchen with loved ones. Acing a basic dish chicken likewise shows kitchen certainty and tolerance, which the best cooks comprehend.

For a formula much praised and cherished, cook chicken ought to be, over all things, straightforward — the meat delicate and succulent, tenderly prepared with salt and scented with herbs. The greater part of your work will be in preparing the chicken for simmering and afterward figuring out how to abide an hour in the kitchen while it cooks.

Refreshing Our Classic Roast Chicken Method

Kitchn first distributed guidelines for a basic dish chicken years prior, and keeping in mind that the strategy is extraordinary, we've discovered that a couple of little changes make for a stunningly better chicken. You'll discover those updates in the formula underneath.

For Your Information

A four-to five-pound chicken is generally alluded to as a grill fryer and will effortlessly serve four to six individuals.

The chicken is done when it registers 165°F in the thickest piece of the thigh. The wings and legs will squirm freely and the juices will run clear.

All out broiling time will be somewhere in the range of one and one-and-a-half hours — the careful cooking time will rely upon the size and sort of your chicken.

5 Steps for Glorious Roasted Chicken

Ensure the chicken is dry: We don't suggest flushing your chicken before broiling. Washing may spread microscopic organisms from the chicken to the sink and crosswise over other nourishment prep surfaces, and we need the chicken's skin to be as dry as could reasonably be expected so it will concoct fresh. When you have the chicken out of its bundling, pat it totally dry all around with paper towels.

Be liberal with the salt: A tablespoon of salt may appear a lot for a little chicken, however you need to be unfathomably liberal with the salt on the skin and inside the chicken's cavity to guarantee that a portion of the flavoring works its way past the skin into the meat. Salting keeps the chicken delicious as well. Oil or margarine on the chicken before broiling is discretionary.

Bracket the chicken: Trussing is a customary strategy for integrating the chicken's legs. Despite the fact that methods for greater poultry like turkey require tying up the entire last part, for a straightforward meal chicken, simply unite the drumsticks with kitchen twine. This extremely just prevents those drumsticks from drying out while the bosom cooks through, and makes the entire chicken cook all the more equally.

Cook with tolerance: A simmered chicken is straightforward, however it isn't fast. The chicken will cook for at least 60 minutes, however you can help the flying creature along by disregarding it. There's no compelling reason to treat or trouble or test the chicken for 60 minutes.

Rest before cutting: Rest the chicken for at any rate 15 minutes before cutting. This enables the chicken to keep on cooking, redistribute its juices, and chill off enough for you to cut it after it rests.

Step by step instructions to Check Chicken Doneness Without a Thermometer

The inquiry we get posed to frequently is "How would I realize my meal chicken is done?" And while a test thermometer is the most ideal approach to decide doneness — it should enroll 165°F in the thickest piece of the thigh before leaving the broiler — there are a couple of different approaches to check.

To start with, adhere to the general standard of 15 minutes for each pound of chicken, a four-pound chicken is going to take at any rate 60 minutes. Second, give the drumsticks a shake; they should squirm effectively. Ultimately, you can embed a knife into the region between the bosom and the thigh, slicing into the meat to watch that the juices are clear (it's ideal to do this test directly out of the stove on the off chance that the chicken needs to return in for more cook time).

Cutting a Roast Chicken

When you're prepared to cut, you'll need a pleasant enormous cutting board and a culinary specialist's knife. I like to begin by expelling the bosom: Make a shallow chop first directly down the focal point of the two bosoms to see the bosom bone. Then, cut between the bosom meat and that issue that remains to be worked out each bosom. Put these in a safe spot.

When the bosom is expelled, you can without much of a stretch evacuate the thighs by flipping the chicken over and pulling up on each. The thigh should pull straight up, yet every so often you'll have to run the knife between the thigh and the spine. Then, lay the chicken thigh level and cut between the thigh and the drumstick at the joint.

You can expel the wings if you like, however I for the most part leave them on and utilize the chicken bones for making stock.

Step by step instructions to Roast a Perfect Chicken

SERVES

4 to 6, contingent upon the size of the chicken

Fixings

1 (4-to 5-pound) entire chicken

Olive oil or softened spread

1 tablespoon genuine salt

Crisply ground dark pepper

Discretionary flavorings: lemon wedges or cuts, new herbs, garlic cloves

Gear

Paper towels

Cooking container, 10-to 12-inch broiler evidence skillet, goulash dish, pie dish, or other ovenproof dish that the chicken fits in

Cutting board

Knife

Kitchen twine

Directions

Preheat the stove to 450°F. Orchestrate a rack in the lower third of the broiler, expel racks above it, and warmth to 450°F. Prepare a work station with your chicken, seasonings, broiling container, and a bit of kitchen twine close by.

Evacuate the giblets. Reach inside the depression of the chicken and evacuate the sack of giblets (if you can't discover them, check in the neck cavity). The giblets can be disposed of, put something aside for stock, or used to make sauce later on.

Pat the chicken dry. Pat the chicken dry with paper towels, making a point to assimilate any fluid behind the wings or legs. Smear inside the body depression as well, getting the chicken as dry as you can all around.

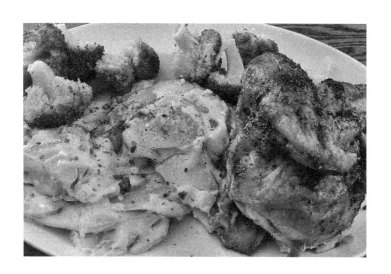

Rub the chicken with olive oil or margarine. Rub a flimsy layer of oil or softened margarine everywhere throughout the chicken, giving uncommon consideration to the bosom and the drumsticks. Be liberal here! The fat will enable the skin to fresh and become brilliant.

Sprinkle liberally with salt and pepper. Sprinkle the chicken done with the salt and pepper. Once more, be liberal here!

Spot flavorings inside the chicken and bracket (discretionary). If wanted, stuff the depression of the chicken with divided lemons, entire cloves of garlic, or herbs. This adds inconspicuous flavor to the chicken. Tie the legs together with a bit of kitchen twine.

Spot the chicken, bosom side up, in the skillet. Spot the chicken bosom side up in a cooking container, cast iron skillet, griddle, preparing dish, pie plate, or some other shallow ovenproof dish. You can cook the chicken independent from anyone else in a skillet, or lift it off the dish utilizing a simmering rack or coarsely slashed vegetables.

Lower the warmth to 400°F and cook for an hour. Spot the chicken in the stove. Quickly lower the broiler temperature to 400°F. Set a clock for an hour and let the chicken meal undisturbed.

Check the chicken. The chicken is done when it registers 165°F in the thickest piece of the thigh, when the wings and legs squirm freely, and when the juices run clear. If the chicken isn't prepared, keep simmering and checking like clockwork until it is finished. Absolute broiling time will be somewhere in the range of 1 and 1/2 hours — careful cooking time will rely upon the size of the chicken.

Rest the chicken. Move the chicken to a perfect cutting board and let it rest for around 15 minutes. During this time, you can prepare a plate of mixed greens or side dish, or whisk some flour into the skillet juices to make sauce.

Cut the chicken. Cut the chicken into the bosoms, thighs, and drumsticks, and serve. Take any outstanding meat out the bones and spare it for different meals.

Formula NOTES

Capacity: Leftovers will keep for around 5 days in the fridge or can be solidified for as long as 3 months.

Flavoring: You can change the kind of the chicken by including a zest rub alongside the salt and pepper. We like Chinese 5-zest mix, za'atar flavors, and ras el hanout.

Simmering with vegetables: You can likewise make a two-in-one meal by broiling the chicken over a bed of potatoes, onions, carrots, or different veggies. Investigate this formula for directions and motivation: Viking Chicken.

THE MOST EFFECTIVE METHOD TO COOK A WHOLE CHICKEN IN THE SLOW COOKER

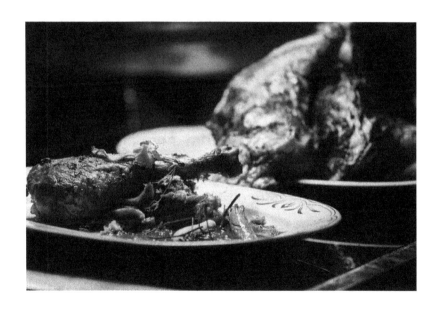

The moderate cooker strikes once more! With insignificant work and only one fixing (psst ... it's chicken) this formula conveys the most scrumptious result comprehensible — meat so delicate and delicious it for all intents and purposes falls directly off the bone. Also, it's everything on account of the little, shut condition of the moderate cooker.

One-Ingredient Slow-Cooker Chicken

The genuine excellence of this formula (indeed, perhaps shockingly better than hands-off cooking!) is the fixing list, as it contains a solitary thing: one entire chicken. OK, you may see salt and pepper on there as well, yet I like to expect those are givens in pretty much every formula. Also, truly, if you want to overlook them, that is fine. The outcome will stun you in any case.

To be completely forthright, I'm normally somewhat questionable of plans that call for only one fixing — with scarcely any info, it's difficult to anticipate a not too bad yield — yet I'm glad to disclose to you that this chicken refutes that conviction completely. It's one of the uncommon occasions only a smidgen of work leaves you with a colossal prize.

Put This Chicken on a Pedestal — Literally

There's one significant advance to remember before adding the chicken to the moderate cooker. You need to make a base for the chicken to lay on with the goal that it's not sitting straightforwardly on the bowl. This could be a little metal rack or trivet (like the one that accompanied your electric weight cooker) or even three to four chunks of aluminum foil — simply enough so the chicken is raised about an inch off the base.

As the chicken cooks, it discharges a decent measure of fluid, more so than simmering in the broiler. Raising the chicken keeps it from sitting in a pool of fluid for an all-inclusive timeframe and furthermore supports more wind stream around the entire winged animal.

If you have a couple of potatoes, carrots, or onions sticking around, feel free to utilize them as a base. Throughout the year, sweet potatoes have gotten a genuine top choice.

Fresh Skin Is Three Minutes Away

While the soggy condition in the moderate cooker makes for genuinely succulent chicken, it has one potential downside: Cooking an entire chicken in the moderate cooker won't give you the sautéed, firm skin you'd get from simmering in the stove. If you're not a skin individual, then this will scarcely matter to you, yet if a feathered creature enveloped by a fresh, crackly skin is the thing you're pursuing, there's a straightforward fix for that.

After the chicken has got done with cooking in the moderate cooker, move it to a heating sheet or dish and pop it under the grill for around three minutes. It's simply sufficient opportunity to change the skin, without warming up your kitchen. Since the chicken is so delicate, it can feel intense to move it out of the moderate cooker, however it's simpler than it appears. I've discovered that the most ideal way is cautiously lifting it utilizing two metal spatulas (fish spatulas are particularly convenient).

The Liquid Gold By-Product

Toward the finish of cooking, you'll notice a decent arrangement of fluid from the chicken in the base of the moderate cooker. This stuff resembles fluid gold, bearing a more extreme and more extravagant flavor than chicken juices. In any case, you'll need to spare and utilize it similarly as you would chicken stock or juices. Keep it in a fixed holder in the cooler for up to a couple of days; generally stash it away in the cooler until you're prepared to utilize it.

The most effective method to Cook a Whole Chicken in the Slow Cooker

SERVES

4 to 6, contingent upon the size of the chicken

Fixings

1 (3-to 4-pound) entire chicken

1 teaspoon legitimate salt

1/2 teaspoon new ground dark pepper

Gear

6-quart moderate cooker or bigger

Metal trivet or aluminum foil

Directions

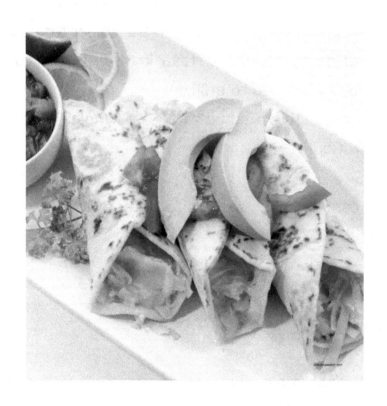

Make a base in the base of the moderate cooker. Spot a little metal rack, heatproof trivet, or three bundles of aluminum foil (each around 3 inches wide) in the bowl of a 6-quart or bigger moderate cooker. This is the base that the chicken will sit over during cooking.

Expel the giblets. Reach inside the pit of the chicken and expel the sack of giblets (if you can't discover them, check in the neck pit). Dispose of them, or spare to make stock or sauce later on.

Pat the chicken dry. Use paper towels to pat the chicken dry. Make a point to retain any fluid behind the wings or legs. Blotch inside the body cavity to get the chicken as dry as would be prudent.

Season the chicken with salt and pepper. Sprinkle the chicken done with the salt and pepper.

Spot the chicken, bosom side up, in the moderate cooker. Spot the entire chicken, bosom side up, over the trivet or chunks of aluminum foil with the goal that it's not sitting on the base of the moderate cooker. Keep the chicken in the focal point of the moderate cooker however much as could be expected.

Cook the chicken. Spread the moderate cooker and cook on the HIGH setting for 2 1/2 to 3 1/2 hours or on the LOW setting for 4 to 5 hours. The definite cooking time will rely upon the size and kind of your chicken.

Check the chicken. The chicken is done when it registers 165°F in the thickest piece of the thigh, when the wings and legs squirm freely, and when the juices run clear.

Sear for fresh skin (discretionary). For extra-firm skin, cautiously move the chicken to a rimmed preparing sheet, broiler safe skillet, or huge heating dish and spot in the stove. Sear for 3 to 5 minutes — just until the skin arrives at your ideal degree of freshness.

Rest the chicken for 15 minutes. When the chicken has got done with cooking, move it to a perfect cutting board. Give it a chance to rest for around 15 minutes before cutting.

Formula NOTES

Capacity: If not utilized quickly, store the cooked chicken in a fixed holder in the fridge for up to 3 to 4 days, or the cooler for as long as 3 months.

3-Ingredient Yogurt Marinated Chicken

Barbecued chicken bosom is a flexible staple that can be transformed into such huge numbers of different meals. Absorb the chicken pieces a citrus and garlic yogurt marinade and you'll have meat that is increasingly delicate and tasty.

3-Ingredient Yogurt Marinated Chicken

Most marinades are basically serving of mixed greens dressings disguising for a section in the fundamental course. Plate of mixed greens style marinades slim as they pull dampness from the meat, so when the meat hits the flame broil, the marinade slips directly off. The arrangement lies in a single unique fixing: yogurt!

Yogurt makes boneless, skinless chicken unendingly progressively delicate, and a yogurt marinade is as simple as one-two-three: one cup of yogurt, two citrus natural products, and three garlic cloves.

Most marinades are basically plate of mixed greens dressings disguising for a section in the fundamental course. Plate of mixed greens style marinades slender as they pull dampness from the meat, so when the meat hits the barbecue, the marinade slips directly off. The arrangement lies in a single unique fixing: yogurt!

Yogurt makes boneless, skinless chicken limitlessly progressively delicate, and a yogurt marinade is as simple as one-two-three: one cup of yogurt, two citrus organic products, and three garlic cloves.

Include Citrus and Garlic for an Easy 3-Ingredient Marinade

Utilize two entire citrus natural products — lemon, lime, or orange — for this tasty marinade. Oranges are better and progressively unpretentious, while lemons and limes are clear and sharp. In spite of the difference in size, pursue the technique beneath regardless of which organic product you pick (and stick to utilizing one kind of citrus).

Get-up-and-go and squeeze one of the citrus natural products for the marinade, then cut the other to flame broil close by the chicken. Finish the marinade with three cloves of garlic, a spot of legitimate salt, and newly ground dark pepper. Do all the prep without a moment's delay, and you won't have to return to the knife square or cutting board. After one nibble of delicate flame broiled chicken and burned citrus, you'll resolve to submit this one to memory.

3-Ingredient Yogurt Marinated Chicken

SERVES

4

PREP TIME:

15 minutes

COOKING TIME:

10 minutes

Fixings

2 medium lemons, limes, or oranges

1 cup plain entire milk yogurt

3 cloves garlic, minced

2 teaspoons legitimate salt

1/2 teaspoon newly ground dark pepper

2 pounds boneless, skinless chicken bosoms or thighs

Directions

If utilizing chicken bosoms, pound dainty first. (There is no compelling reason to pound chicken thighs.) To do as such, place 2 chicken bosoms in a gallon-sized zip-top sack. Utilize the level side of a meat hammer or a moving pin to pound to 1/2-inch thickness. Move the chicken to a plate and rehash with the rest of the bosoms. Ensure your zip-top sack doesn't have any gaps in it from beating the chicken bosoms. If it does, proceed with another sack; generally, make the marinade in a similar pack.

Cut 1 of the citrus natural products into 1/2-inch-thick cuts and refrigerate until prepared to flame broil. Finely grind the pizzazz of the rest of the citrus foods grown from the ground to the sack. Cut the organic product fifty-fifty and crush the juice into the sack. Include the yogurt, garlic, salt, and pepper and mix to join.

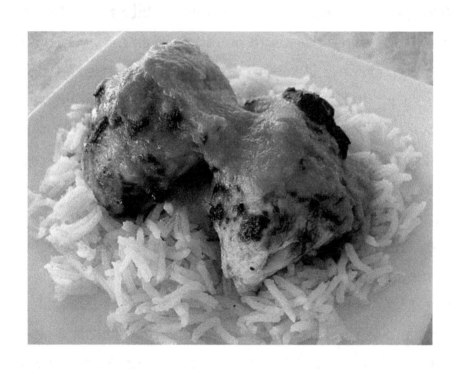

Include the chicken bosoms or thighs, seal the sack, and back rub to cover the chicken with the marinade. Spot the pack on a heating sheet with the goal that the chicken sits level in a solitary layer clinched. Refrigerate for at any rate 30 minutes or medium-term.

When prepared to cook, expel the chicken from the fridge. Prepare an outside barbecue for high, direct warmth. When hot, scratch the flame broil grates if expected to evacuate any waiting coarseness or trash.

Utilizing tongs, expel the chicken from the marinade and spot on the barbecue in a solitary layer. Spread and flame broil undisturbed until barbecue marks show up and the chicken doesn't adhere to the flame broil, around 4 minutes. If it sticks, keep on cooking one more moment until it discharges effectively. Flip and cook the second side until barbecue marks show up and a moment read thermometer embedded into the thickest piece of the chicken registers 165°F, around 5 minutes more. In the mean time, place the held citrus cuts on the flame broil and cook until barbecue marks show up, around 3 minutes for each side.

Move the chicken and citrus cuts to a perfect cutting board. Let rest 5 minutes before cutting the chicken and presenting with the citrus.

Formula NOTES

———

Capacity: Refrigerate remains in a sealed shut compartment for as long as 4 days.

Make ahead: Make the yogurt marinade as long as 2 days ahead of time and store in the icebox.

Stovetop variety: Heat 1 tablespoon of olive oil in a cast iron skillet over medium warmth. Include the chicken (in groups if required) and cook until seared and a moment read thermometer embedded into the thickest piece of the chicken registers 165°F, 6 to 8 minutes for every side.

Instructions to Poach Chicken Breasts

Poaching is one of my go-to meal prep strategies because of its straightforwardness and flexibility. Include aromatics, herbs stems, or citrus strips to the water for additional flavor. Also, in the wake of cooking, cut or shred the chicken to be utilized for servings of mixed greens, sandwiches, bowls, tacos, goulashes, and that's just the beginning.

Oust all musings of stringy, intense, dismal chicken from your brain. For our chicken serving of mixed greens sandwiches and snappy weeknight meals, we don't need anything yet the best. Furthermore, for that, poached chicken is unquestionably the best approach. This technique is simple, quick, and idiot proof. Thoroughly delicate chicken bosoms that are as useful for supper as they are for lunch the following day? Not an issue.

Poached chicken gets some flack for being "diet nourishment," and keeping in mind that the facts demonstrate that poaching chicken requires no fat for cooking and chicken bosoms are normally lean, there are a lot of reasons why poached chicken can remain individually.

Poached chicken is basic for a decent chicken plate of mixed greens (which is undoubtedly not an eating routine nourishment!). When cut, this chicken is additionally an extraordinary include to any verdant green lunch plate of mixed greens or sandwich — route superior to shop meat. This chicken shreds beautifully, so I like utilizing it to make a snappy BBQ pulled chicken or for weeknight tacos. Additionally, come cooler temperatures and meal season, poached chicken is an unquestionable requirement have for a significant number of my preferred prepared suppers.

Poaching chicken is simple. It includes covering chicken pieces with water and giving them a chance to stew on the stovetop until the chicken is cooked through. The low temperature and damp warmth cooking strategy cooks the chicken delicately and keeps it from overcooking too rapidly. The cooked chicken is soggy and delicate — the extremely inverse of intense.

I like boneless, skinless chicken bosoms for this cooking technique, however you can likewise utilize bone-in chicken bosoms or even thighs or drumsticks. The chicken can be cooked with the skin on, yet I like to expel it because the skin doesn't generally include anything with this cooking technique (it's all the more an assistance when simmering or flame broiling). I additionally prefer to strain the poaching fluid and use it for soups and cooking grains, and find that leaving the skin on makes the fluid excessively sleek for my taste.

To knock up the flavor, I include whatever aromatics I have in the kitchen — a cove leave, a couple of crushed garlic cloves, any herbs that need spending. If I have some extra wine or an open container of lager, I'll add a portion of that to the poaching fluid, as well. These will season the chicken as it poaches, making it progressively tasty and enjoyable to eat.

Poached chicken? Amusing to eat? Right on! How would you utilize poached chicken in your cooking?

Step by step instructions to Poach Chicken Breasts

MAKES

1 to 4 chicken bosoms

Fixings

1 to 4 skinless chicken bosoms (bone-in or boneless)

1/2 to 1 teaspoon salt

Aromatics: crushed garlic, narrows leaf, 1 teaspoon peppercorns, cut ginger, new herbs, meagerly cut onions, or some other flavorings

1 cup dry white wine (discretionary)

Hardware

2 to 4-quart sauce pan with cover, sufficiently enormous to hold the chicken bosoms in a solitary layer

Moment read thermometer

Cutting board

Knife

Guidelines

Spot the chicken and aromatics in a pan or pot. Orchestrate the chicken in a solitary layer on the base of the pan or pot enormous enough for them to sit generally in a solitary layer. (It's fine if they cover a bit.) Sprinkle the salt and aromatics over chicken.

Spread the chicken with water. If utilizing wine, pour this over the chicken first. Pour in enough cool water to cover the chicken by an inch or something like that.

Heat the water to the point of boiling. Heat to the point of boiling over medium-high warmth. You'll see some white scummy froth gathering superficially as the water reaches boiling point — if you'll be utilizing the poaching fluid for a soup or other formula, you can skim this off; something else, it's fine to leave it.

Decrease to a stew, spread, and cook. When the water reaches boiling point, lessen the warmth to low, spread the pot, and let the chicken stew. Start checking the chicken following 8 minutes: it is done when misty through the center and a moment read thermometer in the thickest piece of the meat registers 165°F. Chicken will normally get done with cooking in 10 to 14 minutes relying upon the thickness of the meat and whether it is has a bone.

Expel from the poaching fluid. Move the chicken from the poaching fluid to a plate or clean cutting board.

Serve or store the chicken. Poached chicken can be served hot, room temperature, or cool. It can likewise be served entire, or it tends to be cut or destroyed according to your formula. If you cooked your chicken with the bones, you can force or remove the bones, return them to the pot with the poaching fluid, and stew until the fluid is diminished. When stressed, this is a speedy chicken juices that can be utilized for soups or rice.

Formula NOTES

Capacity: Leftover chicken can be put away in a sealed shut compartment in the icebox for as long as 4 days or solidified for as long as 3 months.

Instructions to Make Easy Shredded Chicken in the Slow Cooker

This strategy gives you a similar outcome as poaching chicken on the stovetop, yet proves to be useful when you need something somewhat more uninvolved.

Observe the single nourishment that has changed my week by week meal plan! From tacos to plates of mixed greens to grain bowls, the straightforwardness and flexibility of destroyed chicken truly can't be beat. On account of the moderate cooker and an idiot proof proportion, making a huge amount of destroyed chicken without a moment's delay is conceivable. Here's the way you do it.

Begin with Two Ingredients

It doesn't get a lot simpler or more adaptable than moderate cooker destroyed chicken. It's a set-it-and-overlook it hotshot, and requires only two fixings. Start with boneless, skinless chicken bosoms and your decision of water or chicken stock. I lean toward stock, if I have it convenient, because it includes somewhat more flavor, however water works similarly well. Adding some fluid to the moderate cooker is a fundamental advance, and guarantees that the chicken concocts to be overly delicate and delicious.

The Easy Way to Scale Up or Down

Regardless of whether you're making only a couple of servings or enough to encourage a group, the exertion continues as before. The significant thing to recall is keeping the correct proportion of chicken to fluid.

1/2 cup stock, low-sodium chicken juices, or water for each pound of chicken

Shred Chicken While It's Still Warm

While this method is excessively basic, the chicken doesn't really self-destruct into shreds individually (wouldn't that be decent!). The most significant thing to know is that it's best done when the chicken is still warm, ideally directly after it's finished cooking. Move the meat to a plate or cutting board and utilize two forks to pull it separated. The chicken will be so delicate and delicate that it will for all intents and purposes self-destruct with only a bit of goading.

As the chicken cools, the muscle filaments begin to take care of, which makes it somewhat harder to shred. It's certainly feasible despite everything it works, however it requires some more exertion and the meat will in general draw separated in bigger pieces as opposed to thin, wispy shreds.

Your Solution to a Week of Chicken-Filled Meals

The absolute best thing about concocting a bunch of destroyed chicken is every one of the potential outcomes it brings to mealtime. It can mean seven days of snacks — everything from wraps and burritos to a generous grain bowl garnish to a basic serving of mixed greens are made additionally fulfilling with this protein topper. It's additionally a simple answer for weeknight suppers. When you have a staple like destroyed chicken in the ice chest, the conceivable outcomes are about huge.

The most effective method to Make Easy Shredded Chicken in the Slow Cooker

MAKES

around 4 cups of destroyed chicken

PREP TIME:

5 minutes

COOKING TIME:

2 hours to 5 hours

Fixings

2 pounds boneless, skinless chicken bosoms (around 4)

1 cup chicken stock, low-sodium chicken soup, or water

Gear

Estimating cup

4-quart or bigger moderate cooker

Cutting board or huge plate

Forks

Directions

Add the fixings to the moderate cooker. Spot the chicken and stock, soup, or water in a 4-quart or bigger moderate cooker.

Cook the chicken. Spread and cook until the chicken is delicate and registers an interior temperature of 165°F, 4 to 5 hours on the LOW setting, or 2 to 3 hours on the HIGH setting.

Shred the chicken. Move the chicken to a spotless cutting board or huge plate. While the chicken is still warm, utilize 2 forks to shred the meat. If not utilizing quickly, store the destroyed chicken with a portion of the cooking fluid to keep it sodden.

Formula NOTES

Capacity: Refrigerate the destroyed chicken in a hermetically sealed holder for as long as 4 days or in the cooler for as long as 4 months.

CONCLUSION

You get to the exercise center. You murder your exercises. You receive the rewards of the physical action and love each moment. Be that as it may, do you ever get baffled because you discover the sustenance part of fat loss to be debilitating? Some portion of scares individuals about nourishment prepping that it appears to take up such an extensive amount their leisure time.

You can in any case cook healthy nourishment to keep in your refrigerator, appreciate time with your loved ones, get the chance to take a shot at time, exercise and you won't need to sacrifice anything. When attempting to lose fat or fabricate muscle, having healthy nourishment alternatives available is critical— and it doesn't need to assume control over your life. Truth be told, it should mix directly in.

For the individuals who think eating healthy is excessively costly, reconsider. Meal prepping will set aside you cash because you can purchase things in mass and exploit your cooler. When you put aside time to prep your nourishment, prepare to stun the world regarding volume.

Try not to be frightened to purchase five pounds of chicken rather than one. You can cook each pound in turn if you need to, and solidify the rest so it will consistently be prepared to defrost. You can solidify crisp herbs, prepared egg cups and cooked turkey meatloaf. Continuously load up on staples when they're discounted, for example, olive oil, flavors and mustard. Not exclusively will preparing your very own nourishment set aside you cash; it will spare your waistline also.

Meal prepping is ideal for occupied people. When you get its substance, it will be a non-debatable. Subsequent to causing supper and tidying to up, would you truly like to take everything out again to make lunch? While supper is preparing, pack nourishment for the following day.

This basic errand will assist you with cutting time in the kitchen, and you will feel sorted out and all set for one more day of clean eating. Likewise, don't be reluctant to fill your broiler with different sorts of nourishments on the double. For instance, you can cook two pounds of chicken bosom, three sweet potatoes, broiled vegetables and even eggs at the same time.

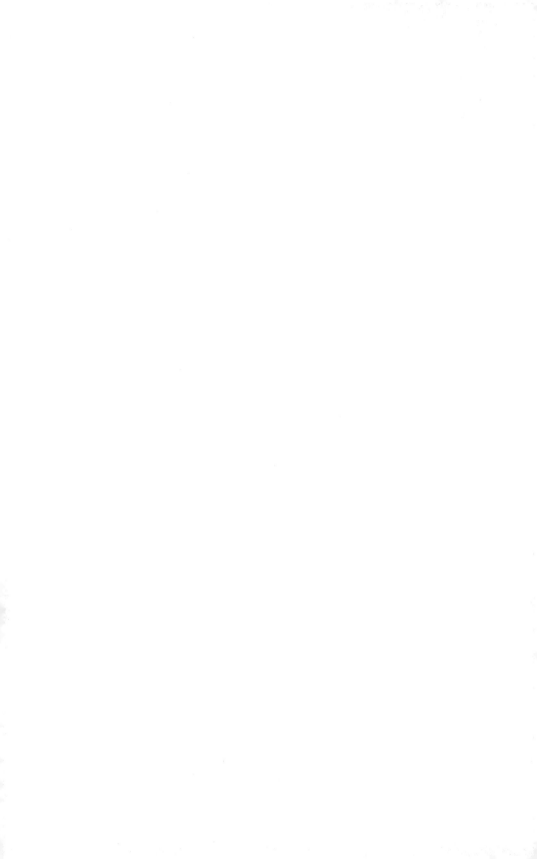